Natural & Herbal Remedies for
Carpal Tunnel Syndrome

Excerpted from *Natural Hand Care,* by Norma Pasekoff Weinberg

CONTENTS

Identifying Carpal Tunnel Syndrome

Carpal tunnel syndrome is an injury commonly associated with repetitive motion. If you spend long hours at your computer terminal, bicycle for long periods of time, are a musician or a factory worker with a high-force, highly repetitious task, or face any other type of repetitive hand-wrist movement or jarring, you may be susceptible to this ailment. The injury usually begins with numbness and tingling or burning in the fingers. It can progress to pain and decreased strength and coordination of the hands and a limited range of motion in the forearm and upper arm. Most cases of carpal tunnel syndrome will resolve on their own or can be treated with natural remedies. In severe cases, however, carpal tunnel syndrome can be crippling, causing muscle atrophy in the thumb and permanent loss of sensation in the fingers. In such cases, surgery is usually recommended.

Carpal tunnel syndrome is caused by undue pressure on the median nerve, which runs through the "tunnel" formed by the carpal bones in the wrist and brings sensation to and assists in the movement of the fingers. High-force repetitive motion, its most well-known cause, can create irritation and inflammation in the carpal tunnel, thus squeezing the median nerve. Bone dislocations or fractures, inflammatory conditions such as rheumatoid arthritis, the fluid retention common to pregnancy, and even hormonal changes caused by menopause can also cause symptoms of carpal tunnel syndrome.

Herbs Will Work, but Use Common Sense

When accompanied by a healthy resting period, a conscious effort to relax your grip, and gentle stretching exercises, herbal remedies can be effective treatments for most cases of carpal tunnel syndrome. However, herbs are never a cure-all, and in more serious cases medical attention from a qualified practitioner may be necessary.

If you're experiencing symptoms of carpal tunnel syndrome, be sure to consult with your primary healthcare provider to ensure that carpal tunnel is the proper diagnosis — tendonitis, for example, can exhibit symptoms similar to those of carpal tunnel syndrome. If you have carpal tunnel syndrome and your symptoms seem to worsen, or if after resting your wrist and trying these natural-care suggestions the symptoms don't improve, ask your primary-care physician for further assistance and recommendations.

Consult a physician for a diagnosis if you experience:
- Recurrent numbness, pain, or a tingling sensation in your fingers, wrist, or hand, especially if it persists at night and if it can be "shaken out"
- A sense of weakness and tendency to drop things
- Loss of feeling of heat or cold
- Persistent feeling of swelling in the hands although no inflammation is visible

Anatomy of the Carpal Tunnel

The carpal tunnel is created by the bones of the wrist, which are laid out in a contour that resembles a shallow basin. There is a narrow opening in the palm side of the wrist made up of eight wrist, or carpal, bones. Three walls of the "tunnel" consist of these carpal bones, while the fourth "wall" is formed by the transverse carpal ligament, a strap of tough ligament.

The carpal tunnel is a very crowded section. The median nerve, which provides feeling for the fingers (except the little finger) and assists in hand and finger movement, and nine tendons that flex the fingers pass through the carpal ligament. As the fingers move and repeat a movement again and again, the area inside the ligament can become irritated, causing the tendons to swell and to squeeze the median nerve. Pressure on the median nerve can cause symptoms of discomfort in the fingers, hand, and elbow. These symptoms may include the sensation of numbness (often most noticeable at night), tingling, burning, cold, pain, and stiffness, or physical problems with grip strength and thumb weakness, depending on how intense the pressure on the nerve is.

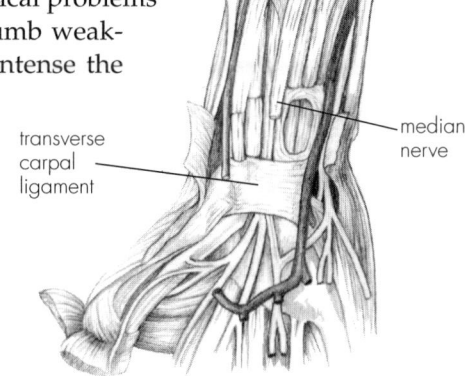

transverse carpal ligament

median nerve

The median nerve runs through the tight space beneath the transverse carpal ligament.

Testing for Carpal Tunnel Syndrome

If you are concerned that you might have carpal tunnel syndrome, there are a couple of simple tests you can perform at home. However, it is important to get an appropriate diagnosis before treating carpal tunnel syndrome, so be sure to see a knowledgeable healthcare professional. More extensive tests include the phenar muscle test, magnetic resonance imaging (MRI), computerized tomography (CT) scans, electromyography (EMG), and nerve conduction studies (NTS).

Tinel's test: This is also known as the median nerve percussion test. Place your hand palm-side up on a table. Tap the area over the median nerve with the index finger of the opposite hand. If you feel tingling or numbness, the test is positive. (Tinel's test is correct in diagnosing carpal tunnel syndrome about 65 percent of the time.)

Phalen's test: Place your elbows on a surface and allow your hands to relax to a 90-degree angle at the wrists. Or gently place the backs of the hands together with no force, and hold this position for 1 minute. If you feel any numbness, tingling, or pain in your thumb, index finger, or ring finger, the test is positive. (Phalen's test is correct in diagnosing carpal tunnel syndrome 75 to 80 percent of the time.)

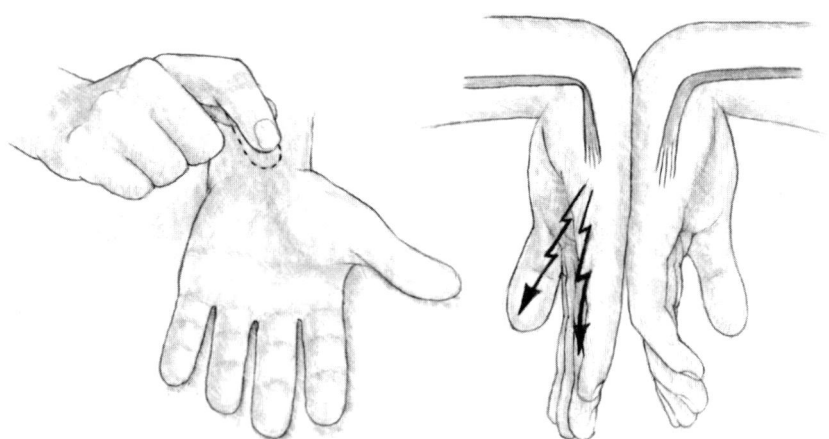

Tinel's test   *Phalen's test*

How Do Joints Work?

A joint is the site where two bones meet and are bound together. The structure of a joint, as well as the way its constituent parts work together, determines the ways in which it can move. A synovial joint such as the wrist is constructed so that only gliding movements are possible. There are six parts to each synovial joint:

Cartilage. The ends of each bone are cushioned and protected by a layer of rubbery connective tissue called cartilage. Feel the central spine of your nose or above the lobe of your ear for a sense of the structure of cartilage. Cartilage has no nerve endings, so cartilage-coated surfaces can make contact without causing pain (or any other sensation). The pain associated with osteoarthritis often results from the wearing away of this cartilage coating in the joints.

Muscles. These elastic tissues stretch and contract to move bones and move us.

Ligaments. Ligaments are short, fibrous bands of tissue that tie bone to bone and enclose the joint capsule.

Tendons. Muscles are attached to the bones by the fibrous tendon cords. You can observe the movement of tendons on the back of your hand.

Synovial membrane. Surrounding each joint site is a synovial sac — a smooth, thin layer of tissue filled with a transparent, egg-white-like fluid. This fluid coats and protects the inner surface of the ligaments and the cartilage that caps the end of the bones.

Bursae. Next to the joint capsule are smaller, fluid-filled lubricating sacs called bursae. Bursae are not always considered components of the joint, but they do serve several important functions: to reduce friction between tendons and ligaments and between tendons and bones; to maintain joint mobility; and to allow the structures to glide freely in relation to each other. Excessive use or injury to a joint can swell these sacs and cause bursitis.

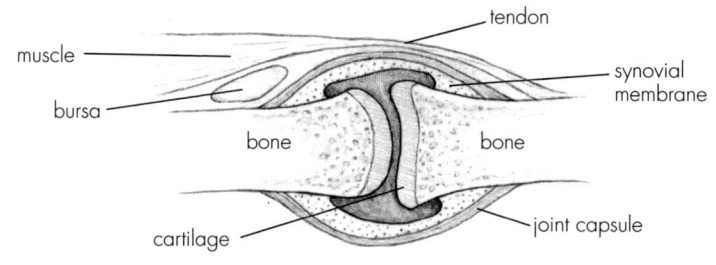

Trigger Finger

Like carpal tunnel syndrome, trigger finger can be caused by repetitive motion; in fact, its symptoms are very similar to those of carpal tunnel syndrome, it is often present in cases of carpal tunnel syndrome, and the two are often confused. For a true diagnosis, you'll need to see a professional. Fortunately, minor cases of trigger finger will benefit equally from treatments and preventive care designed for carpal tunnel syndrome.

A trigger finger results from obstruction of the flexor tendon as a result of repetitive use or trauma to a finger or thumb, which may cause localized swelling of the tendon. This swelling, and the knotlike callus of scar tissue that it may cause as the swollen tendon constantly rubs internally, causes the finger to become stuck as it moves through the space of the A-1 pulley. The A-1 pulley is a structure that holds a tendon close to the bone and normally helps to increase the efficiency of the flexor tendon.

Trigger finger causes jerky movements of the finger and may even cause the finger to become locked in a flexed position. It commonly affects the ring and middle fingers and is four times more prevalent in women than in men. In severe cases, trigger finger may require surgical repair.

Natural treatment for trigger finger focuses on resting the finger from its habitual use. Use cushiony foam grips on pens, pencils, and tools, and at night support the finger with a custom-molded splint on the top finger joint, nearest the fingernail. Try dry brushing to stimulate circulation (see page 27) and daily hand soaks (see the recipe for Dead Sea Salt Hand Baths on page 17) to reduce swelling. To speed healing and reduce scar tissue formation, supplement your diet with vitamin E and zinc.

Computer Wrist Rest

If you spend long hours at the computer, place a small, folded towel at the base of your keyboard or use a premade, commercial padded wrist rest to relieve undue wrist strain.

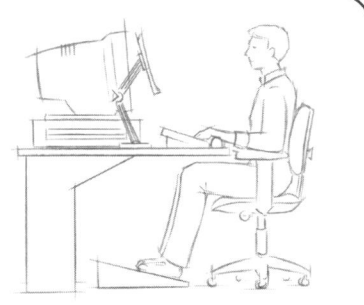

Preventive Care for
Your Hands and Wrists

Whether swinging a tennis racket, playing the guitar, folding an omelet, or typing on a keyboard, human fingers, wrists, arms, and elbows are designed for movement. The undercover structures that allow this ingenious machinery to function include a bony skeleton, tendons, muscles, lubricating membranes, and pliable skin. To allow the movement of which we are capable, each of these structures meets and functions cooperatively at our joints.

Protecting Your Wrist and Fingers

In time, all of us are affected by the stiffness and aches resulting from overuse of our joints. Here are a few suggestions for protecting the joints in your hands and wrists. If you put your mind to it, I'm sure you will be able to think of several more ideas.

- Let your larger joints do the work in place of smaller joints. For instance, carry hangers from the cleaners over your arm and save those finger joints, and instead of carrying a heavy bag or briefcase in your hand, switch to a shoulder strap that transfers the weight to a larger joint.
- Use a food processor or slicing machine instead of a knife (less force on the fingers).
- Use a jar opener to open jars to avoid extra force on the hands and finger joints.
- Use foam padding around a pen or a pencil, a fork, toothbrush, or razor for less joint stress in these everyday tasks.
- Take a break from repetitive tasks, such as computer work, machinery, and bread baking. Gently stretch your hands and arms several times a day. (For stretching exercises, see pages 12–15.)
- When gardening or doing yard work, use the innovative "enabling tools" that are designed to remove stress points from fingers and wrists.

Writer's Cramp

In the *Practical Home Physician* of 1888, under "Diseases of the Nervous System," there is a listing for "writer's cramp." The disorder is described as "a form of paralysis usually limited to certain muscles of the hand . . . common among those whose occupation compels them to hold the pen many hours a day. . . . Writers . . . tailors, and sewing girls who are compelled to use the same muscles constantly for many hours daily are often similarly affected."

With the advent of computer technology and keyboards, it seems we have progressed no further than to electronic writer's cramp — otherwise known as carpal tunnel syndrome. We just can't seem to get ahead!

Rhythmic Finger Exercises

Here are some great finger, hand, and wrist exercises for flexibility, strength, and preventive care that you can do anywhere. This time, no pain equals gain! These exercises will keep your hands limber and strong. If you work in a job at high risk for developing carpal tunnel syndrome, such as a typist or a construction worker using a jackhammer, consider doing these exercises during your breaks to increase circulation to your hands and reduce the risk of inflammation.

This series of exercises is designed and shared by international fitness consultant Barbara Barsham. She claims that a daily dose of these spirited movements will keep your fingers limber and able to do all the finger things you've gotten used to doing!

This is a good warm-up exercise to improve finger-wrist coordination and your mood. No special equipment is needed (except you might want to locate a tape or CD of lively piano music).

Step 1: Thumb-tap. One by one, tap the fingerpads of each finger to the thumb: index to thumb, middle to thumb, ring finger to thumb, and pinkie to thumb, counting 1-2-3-4; then reverse, pinkie to thumb, ring to thumb, middle to thumb, and index to thumb, 4-3-2-1. This should be easy and cause no discomfort. Ten

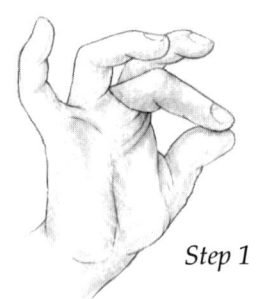

Step 1

times on each hand is a good goal to work toward. Then try both hands at the same time.

Step 2: Thumb-flick. Follow the same procedure, but this time flick each nail off the thumb as if you are flicking off a piece of lint.

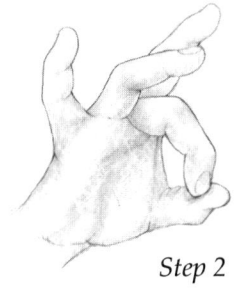

Step 2

Step 3: Finger-palm. With fingers held as straight as possible, touch each one, beginning with your thumb, to your palm in turn, and then reverse and do it again, beginning with your pinkie.

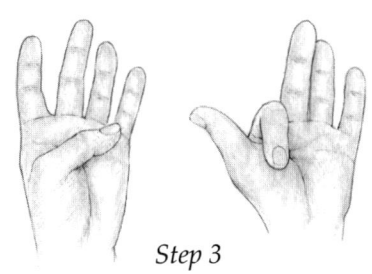

Step 3

Step 4: Piano scales. Pretend there's a piano above your head, almost out of reach. Stretch both hands up above your head and play some five-finger scales on the imaginary piano: C, D, E, F, G — G, F, E, D, C. (For those of you who don't know the scales, pretend you're striking adjacent keys on a piano, one key per finger.) Do this several times. Then bring your hands down to waist level and repeat the procedure, forward and backward.

Last, form your fingers into bent claws and try to play up and down the piano scales again.

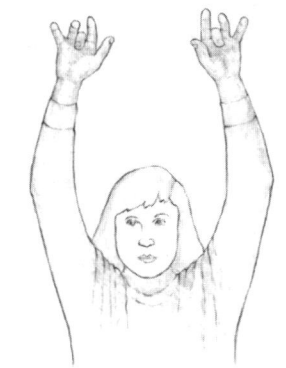

Step 4

Step 5: Finger stretch. With your hands at your sides and your thumbs pointing toward your body, spread your thumbs and fingers as far as they can go and stretch. Hold for a count of 5. Then close them to a fist and hold for a count of 10. Relax. Repeat 10 times.

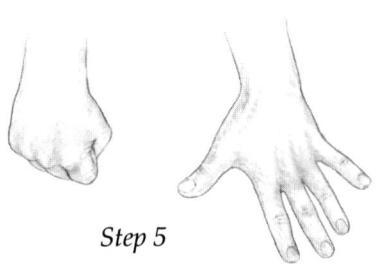

Step 5

Chinese Exercise Balls

Chinese exercise balls are perfectly weighted, hollow, polished chrome or glazed balls that fit comfortably, two at a time, into your palm. They emit a wonderful, delicate chime as they move. The balls are available in different sizes to accommodate large and small hands. To judge the best size for you, hold two balls in a hand. Your fingers should be able to clasp and cover both balls comfortably. You'll find these balls in Eastern gift shops, and they are often available in health food stores.

It's believed that regularly rotating Chinese exercise balls in the palm of each hand not only stimulates the fingers but also taps acupuncture points, improving the circulation of vital energy throughout the body. Use these exercise balls to combat numbness of the fingers and trembling hands, as well as arthritis in the fingers and wrist. Manufacturers of these balls claim that using them "will keep the muscles nimble, the bones strong, the mind sober, the memory intact, relieve fatigue, prevent and cure hypertension, drown your worries, and prolong life." The balls can also be very effective for relaxation and meditation once you get the hang of it. All ages will find them a fun and worthwhile habit.

This exercise calls into motion all the joints of the hand and elbow as well as the muscles of the forearm. It warms the hands and stimulates circulation in the fingers and in the palms of your hands. Begin with your dominant hand and then switch. Start over a table so you won't have to run after the balls as they fall.

Roaring Dragon and Singing Phoenix

Ancient Chinese mandarins believed that palm-size exercise balls induced well-being of the body and serenity of spirit. First hand-forged more than 800 years ago by a blacksmith in Baoding, China, these hollow, iron balls were fashioned with an antique metal soundboard inside. There were two special sounds — one pitched high and the other pitched low — symbolizing yin and yang, and the tones of the roar of the dragon and the song of the phoenix that roamed the grounds of the fabled Yan-Chi Palace. An emperor during the Ming dynasty was so pleased with these balls that he declared them one of the "three treasures" of Baoding.

After you become comfortable with the routine, try doing this exercise daily, while reading or watching television. If you really get into this, you might increase to three or four balls.

Step 1: Put two balls in the palm of your hand. Rotate the balls in a clockwise direction using your thumb and all the fingers as guides. Try to work up a regular, smooth rhythm over several minutes before switching to the reverse direction.

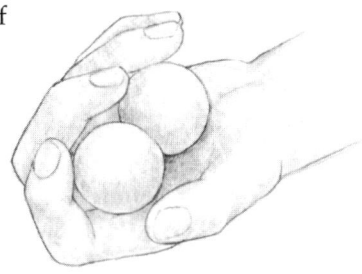

Step 2: Reverse direction and go counterclockwise. This is a larger challenge for the fingers and brain.

Use your fingers and thumb to rotate the balls in a circular motion on your palm.

Treating Carpal Tunnel Syndrome

The traditional treatment for carpal tunnel syndrome focuses on:
- Rest, which reduces irritation and thus inflammation
- Decreasing inflammation to release pressure on the median nerve
- Increasing circulation to the area to promote faster healing

Gentle stretching exercises and vitamin B_6 have also been shown to offer relief.

Rest

Once diagnosed with carpal tunnel syndrome, or when you begin to experience pain in your fingers or wrists, the best thing you can do for yourself is to rest your hands. The inflammation that causes carpal tunnel will not subside without rest, so avoid any activities that could aggravate the condition for at least 2 weeks. In some cases, your healthcare provider may suggest wearing a brace or wrist support at night. The brace will hold your wrist in a relaxed position, neither too flexed nor too bent, which will open up the carpal tunnel and keep you from unintentionally aggravating the condition while you sleep.

Stretching for Relief

Specially designed soft, slow, gentle stretching exercises can bring relief to those with carpal tunnel or other repetitive strain injuries. Sharon Butler, in *Conquering Carpal Tunnel,* talks about the concept of a "stretch point." This is the first hint of a stretch, a slight resistance to the movement. It will appear at the beginning of the stretch and fade as the tissue releases. This loosening is the beginning of change and of healing. She suggests that it helps to close your eyes when practicing stretching exercises. For each of these exercises, start with one set of 10 repetitions and build up to three sets of 10 each time.

GENTLE WRIST FLEX

Step 1: Extend one arm in front of you with your palm and fingers facing up.

Step 2: Take the other hand and place it sideways across the outstretched palm, as in reaching for a handshake.

Step 3: Press gently against the palm and the fingers for a mild extension. Repeat on the opposite side. This is an easy and important stretch to do when you are spending a lot of time sitting in front of a computer.

Step 4: For this slightly more vigorous stretch, hang your hand, palm-side down, over a shelf, table, or armchair. Use your other hand to bend it down as far as comfortably possible. Repeat with the opposite hand.

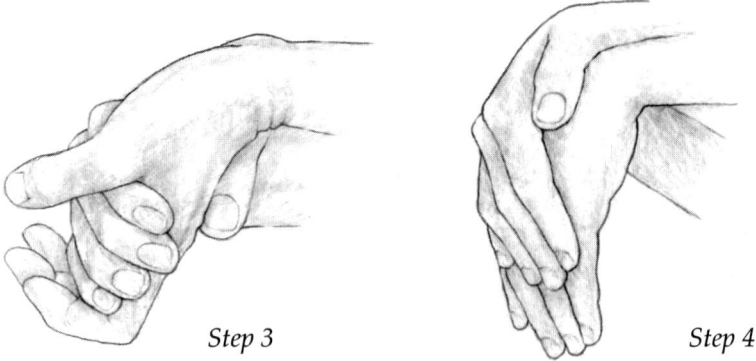

Step 3   *Step 4*

DADDY LONGLEGS HANDSTAND

You can do this exercise seated at a table or walking your hand up a wall.

Step 1: Begin with the palm and fingers flat on the surface.

Step 2: Put gentle pressure on the thumb and little finger and raise the hand up on all the fingers, like a daddy longlegs. Hold and count to 5, and slowly slide back down. Repeat with each hand five times as long as there is no pain.

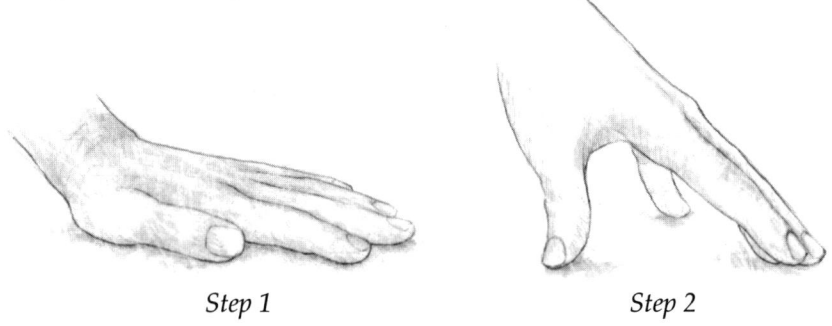

Step 1   *Step 2*

WINDSHIELD WIPER HANDS

This is an easy wrist stretch. It may be a windshield wiper experience, but let's hope you will have a sunny day!

Step 1: Sit down and rest one arm on a table. Move one hand as a windshield wiper would function, side to side, toward the thumb and then away from the thumb. Do 10 repetitions in each direction. Repeat with the other hand.

Step 2: Place both forearms on the table. Lift at the wrist and bring index fingers together and then apart. Continue inward, outward.

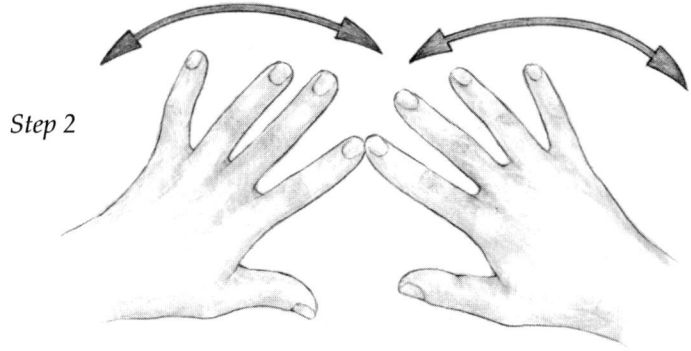

Step 2

WISHING POSE PRESS

Step 1: Put both hands together, with your palms touching and fingers interlaced.

Step 2: Pressing the palms, push the right hand backward with the force of the left.

Step 3: Reverse, pushing the left hand backward with the strength of the right. The pressure should emanate from the palms, not the fingers. Bend just till the feeling of discomfort.

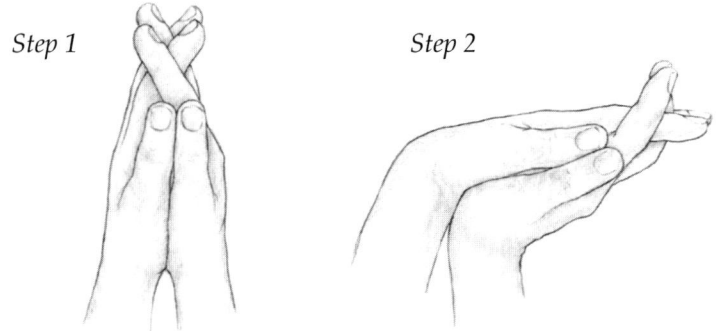

Step 1   *Step 2*

WINGS WRIST STRETCH

Step 1: Place your palms together in front of your chest, fingers pointed up.

Step 2: Keeping palms together, slowly raise elbows up as far as possible without discomfort. Release. Repeat slowly.

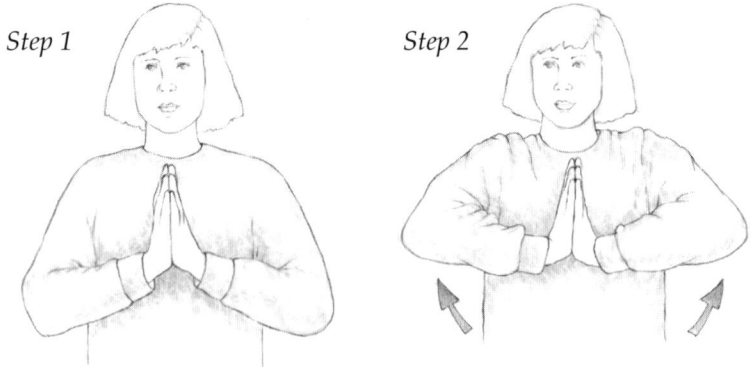

Step 1   *Step 2*

FAR EAST WRIST STRETCH

A gentle, isometric stretch for wrists and fingers, this exercise provides elements of stretching, flexing, and range of motion.

Step 1: Place your hands together with the fingers pointing upward in a prayer position or in a hand position you might see as a welcoming greeting if you visited the Far East.

Step 2: Extend your thumbs in a right angle from your fingers. Keep your fingers together.

Step 3: Now, open and spread your fingers while slowly pushing fingertip against fingertip. Extend your fingers as far apart as you can and still be comfortable. It will look as if you are forming a miniature temple with your hands. Hold with gentle pressure, as if you were doing isometrics, for a count of 10.

Step 4: Relax back to a closed-fingers-and-thumb position.

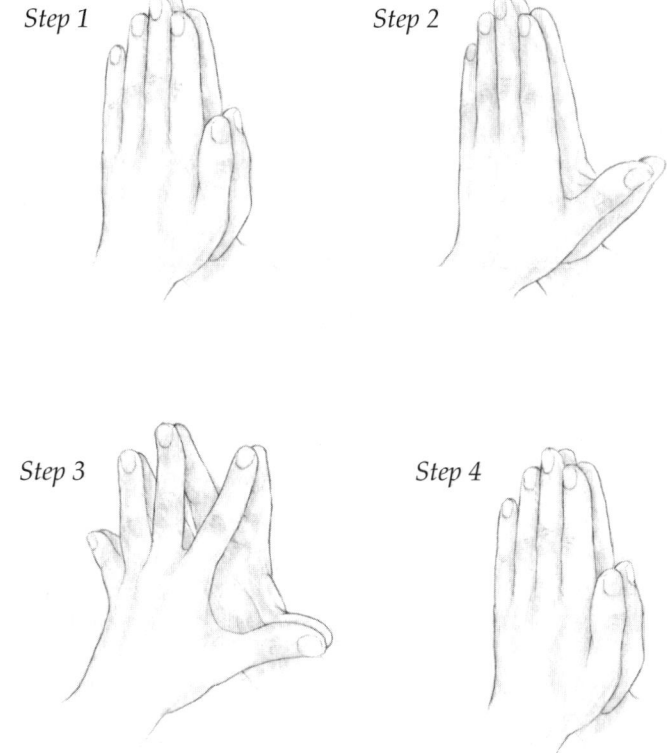

Step 1

Step 2

Step 3

Step 4

Vitamin Therapy

Vitamin B_6 supplementation has been shown to provide some relief to persons suffering from carpal tunnel syndrome and other repetitive-motion injuries. As a daily supplement, take 10 mg; for a short-term therapeutic dosage, take 50 to 200 mg (but be sure to check with your primary healthcare provider before self-medicating). Take B_6 as a supplement early in the day, as it may cause intense dreams and restlessness if taken at night. Natural sources of B_6 include meats, whole grains, brewer's yeast, legumes, potatoes, carrots, eggs, and bananas.

BREAKFAST BOOST

From *Naturally Healthy Skin*, by Stephanie Tourles (Storey Books, 1999)

This recipe is loaded with B vitamins, calcium, potassium, zinc, iron, fiber, protein, and complex carbohydrates for sustained energy. In addition to providing your body with ample amounts of B_6, it's also great for reducing stress and will do wonders for your complexion!

1	frozen banana
2	cups (500 ml) low-fat milk or fortified soy milk
1	tablespoon (15 ml) brewer's yeast
2	teaspoons (10 ml) blackstrap molasses
2	teaspoons (10 ml) raw sunflower seeds
1	teaspoon (5 ml) raw sesame seeds
10	raw almonds
¼	cup (60 ml) raw or cooked oatmeal
2	teaspoons (10 ml) honey
¼	teaspoon (1 ml) ground cinnamon
2–3	ice cubes (optional — makes a thick, frosty drink)

To make:

Combine all the ingredients in a blender and whiz on high until smooth, 30 to 60 seconds total.

To use:

You can consume the entire batch as a breakfast meal or pour half the recipe into a mug and refrigerate the rest until later in the day.

MAKES APPROXIMATELY TWO 1½-CUP (375 ML) SERVINGS
OR 1 LARGE MEAL

Herbal Treatments

These herbal remedies have been formulated to decrease inflammation, increase circulation, and relieve pain. Experiment with the different recipes to find the ones that offer the most relief for your particular condition.

DEAD SEA SALT HAND BATH

This is a helpful soak suitable for all types of overuse injuries, including carpal tunnel syndrome and trigger finger. Dead Sea salts are warming and relaxing.

- 2   quarts (2 liters) boiling water
- 1   teaspoon (5 ml) Dead Sea bath salts
- ⅔   teaspoon (3 ml) Epsom salts
- ⅓   teaspoon (2 ml) baking soda
- 2   drops essential oil of your choice: lavender, juniper, cypress, rosemary, or grapefruit

To make:

1. Pour the boiling water into a large, deep ceramic or glass bowl.

2. Add the Dead Sea salts, Epsom salts, and baking soda. Stir to dissolve. Stir in the essential oil.

To use:

When the water has reached a comfortable temperature, soak the affected hand and wrist for 5 to 10 minutes, or until the water feels cool.

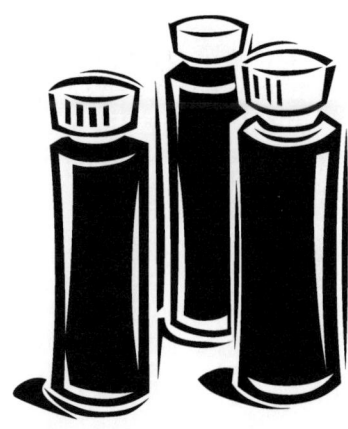

PARAFFIN HAND BATH

Paraffin is a waxy substance that holds in heat. This causes the pores to open and allows moisturizers and healing herbs to penetrate the skin. St.-John's-wort, chamomile, marjoram, and lavender have anti-inflammatory properties. After this treatment, your hands and wrists will feel soft and more comfortably flexible.

> **4 ounces (115 g, or 1 block) paraffin wax**
> **1 ounce (30 ml) olive, almond, or avocado oil**
> **20 drops (1 ml) essential oil of chamomile, marjoram, or lavender**
> **A few drops of St.-John's-wort oil (see recipe on page 22) or carrot seed oil (enough to coat your hands)**

To make:

1. Slowly heat the paraffin, the olive, almond, or avocado oil, and the essential oil in the top part of a double boiler until the paraffin has melted. (Never heat wax directly over an open flame or burner, and never leave wax unattended.)

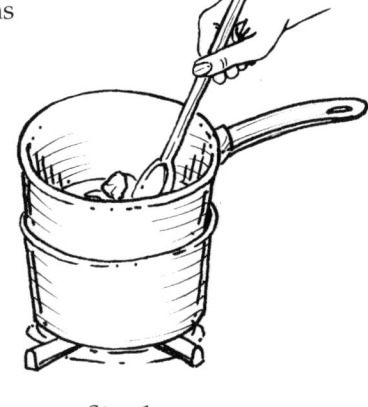

2. Lightly grease a pie plate or a large glass or ceramic casserole with olive oil (the oil coating will make the plate easier to clean later). The vessel should be large enough to accommodate your hand and wrist.

Step 1

3. Carefully pour the melted paraffin and oil mixture into the pie plate or casserole. When a thin skin forms on the surface of the wax, the temperature should be right for dipping the hand. Test the wax mixture for temperature comfort with a drop of wax on the inside of your wrist.

To use:

1. While waiting for the mixture to cool, wash your hand and wrist and pat dry. Completely coat your hand and wrist with the St.-John's-wort oil.

2. Dip your hand and wrist repeatedly into the melted paraffin mixture to build up wax layers. The heat and oil will penetrate the muscles and tendons and help relieve stiffness and pain as well as hydrate the skin.

3. Slide your hand inside a zip-seal plastic bag — you may require some assistance with this step. Cover your hand with a towel and relax for 15 to 20 minutes.

4. When the time is up, peel away the wax by grasping the paraffin-covered hand above the wrist and pulling down. The wax should come off in large pieces. Keep your hand in the plastic bag as you peel away the paraffin to catch all the pieces of wax.

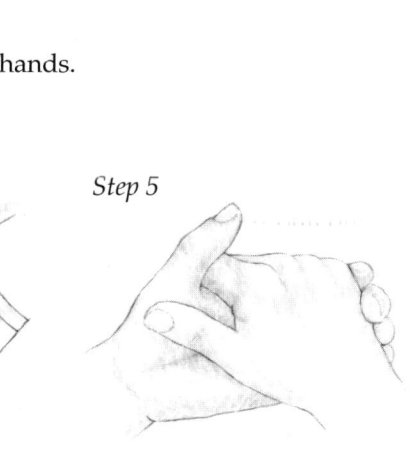

Step 3

5. Massage and gently stretch your hands.

Step 4

Step 5

GINGER WARMING COMPRESS

Ginger is a natural circulatory stimulant and an anti-inflammatory herb that has been used for centuries, both internally and externally, in folk medicine. This warming compress will help to relieve pain.

>**1 piece fresh gingerroot**
>**2 quarts (2 liters) boiling water**
>**St.-John's-wort oil (optional; see recipe on page 22)**

To make:

1. Grate fresh gingerroot and tie it in cheesecloth.

2. Put the ginger into the boiling water. Reduce heat and simmer for 30 minutes.

3. Cool to a warm but comfortable temperature.

To use:

1. If the skin on your hands and wrists is very sensitive, apply a thin layer of St.-John's-wort oil to the area around the wrist before you apply the compress.

2. Remove the cheesecloth with the ginger-root. Dip a clean hand towel into the ginger water. Wring out the excess liquid and apply the comfortably warm cloth to the tender wrist area.

3. Cover with a dry towel to insulate the heat.

4. Rewarm every 5 minutes, as desired.

Ginger
(Zingiber officinale)

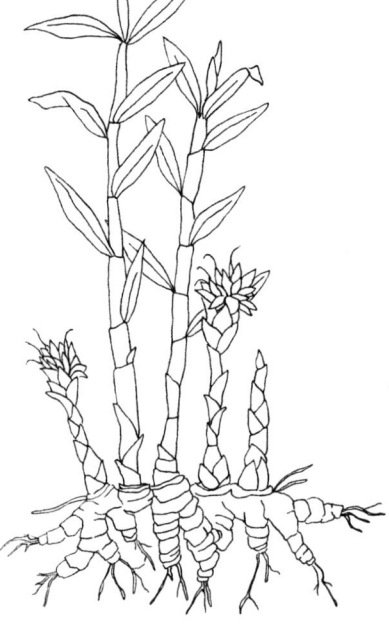

FLEXIBILITY TEA

From *Herbal Teas,* by Kathleen Brown (Storey Books, 1999)

This nutrient-rich blend helps nourish the ligaments, bones, joints, and tendons. In addition to soothing away the inflammation associated with carpal tunnel syndrome, it's also a great recipe for those recovering from sports injuries and for pre- and post-surgery.

2	parts oatstraw
2	parts horsetail
1	part alfalfa leaves
1	part hawthorn berries, crushed
1	part red clover blossoms
1	part rose hips (organic)
¼	part orange slices (organic)

To make:

Combine all the herbs in a pot and cover with boiling water, using 1 quart (1 liter) of water per ounce (28 g) of herbs. Stir well, cover, and let steep 15 to 20 minutes.

To use:

Drink up to 4 cups (1 liter) per day, hot or iced.

ANTI-INFLAMMATORY TEA

This recipe was originally formulated for treating arthritis but will also work well for carpal tunnel syndrome. Devil's claw, a native of the Kalahari Desert, has anti-inflammatory and mild analgesic properties with a cortisone-like action for stiff joints. Celery seed helps to counter acid in the blood.

½–1	teaspoon (2.5–5 ml) dried rhizome of devil's claw, crushed
1	teaspoon (5 ml) celery seed
1	cup (250 ml) spring water

To make:

Stir the herbs into the water. Bring to a boil, cover, and let simmer for 15 minutes. Strain.

To use:

Drink 2 cups a day. Keep it up for at least a month to judge if the tea is effective in reducing pain.

Caution: This tea is not suggested for pregnant or nursing women or those suffering from gastric or duodenal ulcers.

ST.-JOHN'S-WORT OIL

St.-John's-wort (Hypericum perforatum*) is a sun-loving plant that grows easily in many parts of the world and can be cultivated in your own backyard. The oil made from its flower heads has both analgesic and antiseptic properties and can be used topically to encourage healing of cuts, scratches, and minor burns, to ease stiffness of inflamed joints, and to soothe nerve pain. You can often buy St.-John's-wort oil in herb shops, or you can make your own at home by following these simple steps.*

Fresh flower heads of St.-John's-wort
Cold-pressed olive oil to cover

To collect the flowers:

1. Collect just the top 2 inches (5 cm) of the flowering heads of this plant (some purists collect only the just-opening flower heads). Shake out the flowers as you pick, to leave any residents in their home location.

2. You'll need to wilt the flowers so that a large proportion of the water they contain can evaporate, maximizing the potency of the preparation they'll be used in. To wilt freshly picked flowers, spread them in a single layer onto an herb-drying screen or lay them on newspaper that's covered with paper towels. Keep the flowers in a place that has plenty of air circulation but that is out of the sun and away from dust and dirt. After 24 hours, the flowers should be nicely wilted and most of the water they contain should have evaporated.

St.-John's-wort
(Hypericum perforatum)

To make the oil:

1. Fill a clean, dry, widemouthed mason jar to the top, loosely packed, with the freshly wilted flowers. Bruise the petals with a wooden spoon. Cover with olive oil.

2. Stir with a non-metal utensil (such as a wooden chopstick) to release any trapped air bubbles and to allow the oil to penetrate the crevices of the flowers. Top off with more oil, seal, and label.

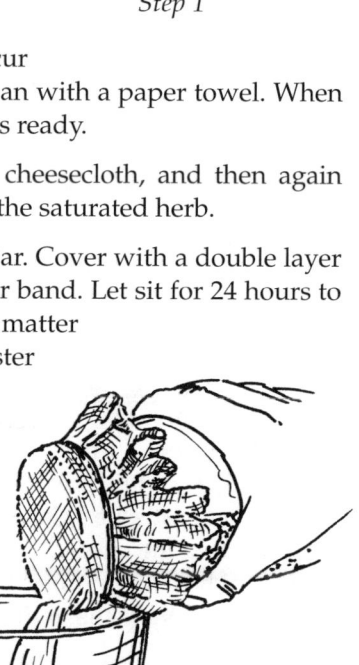

Step 1

3. Set the sealed jar in direct sunlight, turning every day. Keep an eye out for possible mold that may occur inside the jar, and if it does, wipe it clean with a paper towel. When the oil has turned red (3 to 4 weeks), it's ready.

4. Filter the oil through a fine mesh cheesecloth, and then again through a paper coffee filter. Compost the saturated herb.

5. Pour the filtered red oil into a clean jar. Cover with a double layer of cheesecloth and secure with a rubber band. Let sit for 24 hours to observe. If any sludge or particulate matter settles to the bottom, use a poultry baster to transfer the top oil into another clean jar. Seal, label, and date. Store the oil in the refrigerator, where it will keep for up to 6 months.

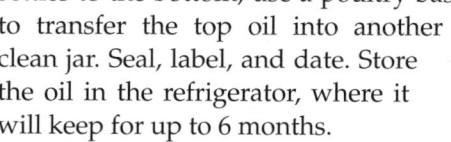

Step 6

CARAMEL CUBES

You can use this wonderful, warming remedy, contributed by herbalist Donna Wood Eaton of Cedar Spring Herb Farm on Cape Cod, Massachusetts, for spot treatment of pain and inflammation caused by carpal tunnel syndrome, trigger finger, osteoarthritis, or rheumatoid arthritis. Cayenne peppers contain aspirin-like ingredients and stimulate the body to release pain-relieving chemicals called endorphins.

8	**ounces (225 g) beeswax**
2	**fresh cayenne peppers, or 1 dried**
60	**drops (3 ml) St.-John's-wort oil (see recipe on page 22)**

To make:

1. Melt the beeswax and toss in the cayenne pepper. Simmer slowly for 10 minutes, then remove the pepper.

2. Add the St.-John's-wort oil and stir to blend. Pour the mixture, while still warm, into empty ice-cube trays.

3. Freeze the cubes and then transfer them to heavy-duty freezer bags. Label and store in the freezer.

To use:

1. Melt a cube in a small, old, stainless-steel pot.

2. Have toilet tissue and a pastry brush at hand. As the beeswax mixture melts, lay the tissue in the palm of your hand and paint the wax onto strips of the tissue. Quickly apply around the affected joint. To retain heat after applying the beeswax, wrap the entire joint in plastic wrap.

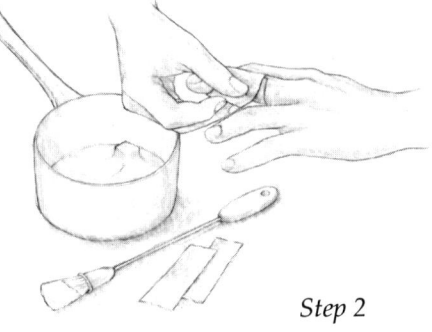

Step 2

3. Allow the beeswax mixture to remain on the area for at least 20 minutes. Repeat at least three times a week to lessen the pain and stiffness of affected joints.

Caution: Fair-skinned folks may find that the skin under the wax turns very red. If this is the case, first coat the area with olive or almond oil. If it continues to irritate the skin, discontinue treatment.

ARNICA COMPRESS

This is a soothing herbal remedy that is effective on all types of inflammatory conditions, including sprains, bruises, and carpal tunnel syndrome. Both St.-John's-wort oil and arnica extract are worth having in your home or travel first-aid kit.

A handful of burdock leaves or green cabbage leaves
2 cups (500 ml) boiling water
1–4 teaspoons (5–20 ml) arnica extract
2 cups (500 ml) hot water
St.-John's-wort oil (see recipe on page 22)
Wide gauze

To make:

1. Pound the fresh burdock or cabbage leaves, then immerse them in boiling water for 2 minutes. Drain the leaves on paper towels.

2. Combine the arnica extract and hot water.

To use:

1. Coat the skin of the affected area with St.-John's-wort oil.

2. Dip a soft, thin towel in the warm arnica wash. Squeeze out the excess liquid and apply the towel to the affected area.

3. Cover with warm, wilted burdock or cabbage leaves.

4. Wrap with wide gauze to hold the compress in place. Repeat twice a day until the swelling has subsided.

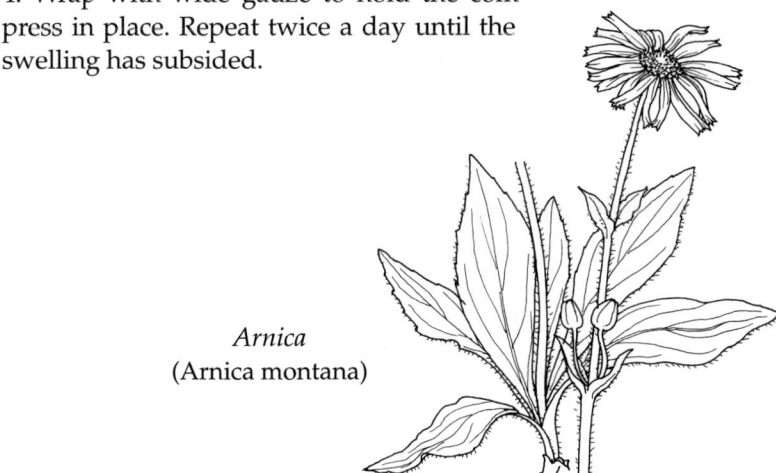

Arnica
(Arnica montana)

SOOTHING HERBAL POULTICE

From *Natural Foot Care*, by Stephanie Tourles (Storey Books, 1998)

This is another herbal recipe that was originally formulated as a treatment for arthritis, but it can work wonders for the pain and inflammation of carpal tunnel syndrome as well. Based on several formulas that were used over a century ago, this poultice revs up the circulation and helps ease stiffness and pain. All herbs called for are in dry form.

- 2 tablespoons (30 ml) plantain leaves
- 3 tablespoons (45 ml) powdered marsh mallow root
- 1 tablespoon (15 ml) powdered meadowsweet leaves
- 1 teaspoon (5 ml) powdered cayenne pepper

To make:

1. Combine all the ingredients in a medium-size bowl.

2. Add enough boiling water to form a paste. Stir until the mixture reaches a gooey consistency and feels slippery. Allow to cool a bit if the paste is too hot to touch comfortably.

To use:

1. Spread the paste on a piece of flannel and place over the swollen joint. Wrap the area with plastic wrap. Cover with a warm towel — right out of the dryer, if that's possible. Sit in a comfortable chair, elevate your wrist, and relax for 30 minutes or longer.

2. When finished, rinse your wrist and apply a thick moisturizing cream to both the hand and forearm.

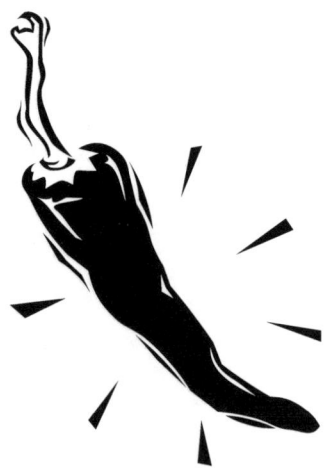

Dry Brushing

Popular in northern Europe, skin brushing with a dry loofah or soft, natural-bristle brush is an invigorating way to slough off dead skin and stimulate circulation. You can brush yourself or make it a mutual experience. To brush the skin of your hands, use a light touch and circling movements in a brisk, flicking, upward direction. Begin with brushing the fingers, then move up the hands to the arms, always brushing toward the heart. Choose the firmness of the brush according to your skin type. The more fragile your skin, the more gentle the brush should be.

A natural sponge gourd *(Luffa cylindrica)* is generally a good choice for dry brushing. A tropical plant native to Asia and Africa, its fruit fibers remain after the fruit has decayed and are uncommonly resistant to molds even when they are continually kept wet.

Caution: Do not practice dry brushing on areas affected by rashes, eczema, or psoriasis.

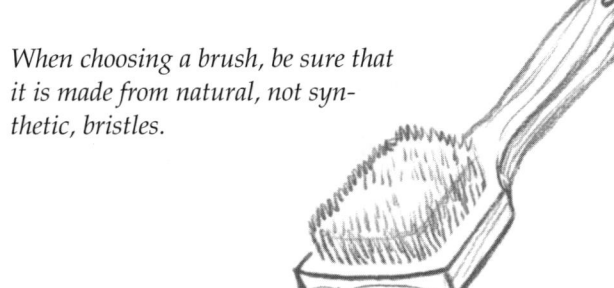

A loofah sponge is the fibrous core of the Luffa cylindrica *gourd; it makes a wonderful natural exfoliating tool.*

When choosing a brush, be sure that it is made from natural, not synthetic, bristles.

Hand Massage

Gentle hand massage can both relieve pain and increase circulation to the affected area. For people suffering from carpal tunnel syndrome, the key word is *gentle*. You don't want to aggravate the condition by irritating the already inflamed area.

These strokes are adapted from those suggested by Michael Reed Gach, author of *Arthritis Relief at Your Fingertips*.

Moisturize. Rub on a moisturizing cream or 1 tablespoon (15 ml) of slightly warmed avocado oil mixed with 3 to 5 drops of your favorite essential oil.

Palm rub. Rub your palms together briskly to create some warmth, then rub the backs of each hand.

Back of hands press. Clasp the fingers of both hands together with the palms facing. Squeeze the fingertips against the back of your hands. Hold for 5 to 10 seconds. Relax. Breathe deeply. Repeat.

Web pinch. The space between each of your fingers is the web. Pinch between the thumb and the index finger, hold for a moment, then rub. Repeat this process between each of the fingers on both hands. Eastern therapies hold that applying pressure on the finger's web site (not the Internet!) helps to dispel headaches and move toxins from the body.

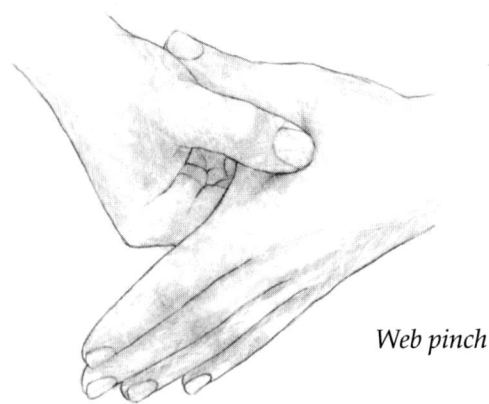

Web pinch

Finger circles. Use your opposite hand to gently stretch and make little circles with each finger and thumb. Reverse direction of finger rotation. Repeat on the other hand.

Wrist compress. Support the wrist of one hand with the palm, fingers, and thumb of the other and squeeze lightly for about 5 seconds. Next, gently rock back and forth the wrist being held in the grasp of the supporting hand, while gently moving the holding hand in the opposite direction. Give the other wrist the same gentle treatment.

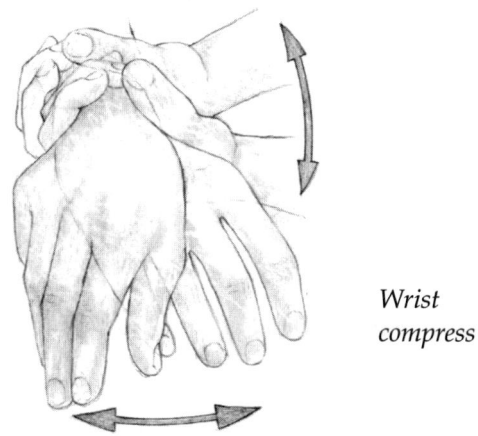

Wrist compress

Forearm press. Knead the outer muscle of the forearm below the elbow. Push the tips of your four fingers sensitively into the skin, using the thumb as an anchor, and work slowly up and down the arm, about three times, as if you were kneading bread dough. Repeat on the other arm.

Elbow rub. Moisturize the elbow and forearm with your cream or avocado oil mixture by massaging with the fingertips of the opposite hand in circular movements from the elbow down to the wrist, then over the hand and fingers.

Arm and finger stretch. Interlace the fingers of both hands with the palms facing and then slowly turn the palms outward. Stretch your arms in front of you and give the fingers and arms an easy, relaxed stretch. Release and gently shake out your hands.

Resources

Mail-Order Sources of Herbs and Herbal Supplies

Aromatherapy International
3 Seal Harbor Road, #735
Winthrop, MA 02152
(800) 722-4377
Fax: (617) 846-5474
Web site: www.aromausa.com
Quality essential oils.

Aubrey Organics
4419 N. Manhattan Avenue
Tampa, FL 33614
(800) 282-7394
Fax: (813) 876-8166
*A variety of natural preparations.
Many of their products are carried
nationwide in natural food stores.*

Dry Creek Herb Farm
13935 Dry Creek Road
Auburn, CA 95602
(530) 878-2441
*A variety of organic and wildcrafted
herbs and herbal preparations.*

Frontier Cooperative Herbs
3021 78th Street
P.O. Box 299
Norway, IA 52318
(800) 669-3275
Fax: (800) 717-4372
*Organic and wildcrafted bulk herbs
and herbal products.*

Herbs 'n Honey
281 Monson Road
Stafford Springs, CT 06076
(860) 684-0551
*Beeswax, honey ointment, cleansing
grains, and more.*

Jean's Greens Herbal Tea Works
119 Sulphur Springs Road
Norway, NY 13416
(315) 845-6500
Fax: (315) 845-6501
Web site: www.jeansgreens.com
*Herbal teas, bulk herbs and spices,
herbal supplies.*

Liberty Natural Products
8120 SE Stark Street
Portland, OR 97215
(503) 256-1227
*Offers a variety of herbal extracts, es-
sential oils, and natural products.*

Mountain Rose Herbs
20818 High Street
North San Juan, CA 95960
(800) 879-3337
Fax: (530) 292-9138
*Organically grown herbs, cosmetic
ingredients, bottles.*

Sage Woman Herbs™
406-B South 8th Street
Colorado Springs, CO 80904
(888) 350-3911
Fax: (719) 473-8873
Quality herbs and herbal preparations.

Rehabilitation Supplies

Sammons Preston
Enrichment Program
Priority Code C50
P.O. Box 5071
Bolingbrook, IL 60440-9973
(800) 323-5547
In-depth catalog featuring aids for daily living and orthopedic supplies for those with conditions that impact hand movements; source for arthritis elbow supports, ergonomic canes, soft-touch scissors, thumb and wrist supports, ergonomic pens, and hand-friendly kitchen and garden tools.

Helpful Organizations

American Association of Naturopathic Physicians
601 Valley Street, Suite 105
Seattle, WA 98109
(206) 298-0126
Provides referrals to national network of naturopathic practitioners.

The American Occupational Therapy Association
4720 Montgomery Lane
P.O. Box 31220
Bethesda, MD 20824-1220
(301) 652-2682
Fax: (301) 652-771
Web site: www.aota.org
Booklets on home rehabilitation exercises and carpal tunnel syndrome.

American Society of Hand Therapists (ASHT)
401 North Michigan Avenue
Chicago, IL 60611-4267
(312) 321-6866
Fax: (312) 527-6866
Has a database of qualified hand therapists; publishes The Journal of Hand Therapy.

International Hand Research Library
100 East Liberty Street, Suite 100
Louisville, KY 40202
(800) 361-9965
Web site: www.handlibrary.org
A nonprofit library serving as a globally accessible, comprehensive resource for all scientific, medical, and general information related to the hand.

Other Storey Books You May Enjoy

Natural Hand Care: Herbal Treatments and Simple Techniques for Healthy Hands and Nails, by Norma Pasekoff Weinberg. Focusing on alternative and preventive therapies and treatments for healthy hands, this book offers dozens of easy-to-make recipes, nutritional advice, strength-building exercises, and relaxing hand-massage techniques. Paperback. 272 pages. ISBN 1-58017-053-6.

Natural Foot Care: Herbal Treatments, Massage, and Exercises for Healthy Feet, by Stephanie Tourles. From easy-to-make recipes for creams, lotions, and ointments to foot-massage techniques, this book offers dozens of natural ways to care for feet. Readers will also find tips for choosing properly fitting shoes and advice for treating athlete's foot and other common foot maladies. Paperback. 192 pages. ISBN 1-58017-054-4.

Naturally Healthy Skin: Tips & Techniques for a Lifetime of Radiant Skin, by Stephanie Tourles. This hands-on guide includes dozens of healing recipes and effective solutions to common skin problems, including acne, age spots, dermatitis, eczema, hives, psoriasis, and sunburn. Paperback. 208 pages. ISBN 1-58017-130-3.

Herbal Teas: 101 Nourishing Blends for Daily Health & Vitality, by Kathleen Brown and Jeanine Pollack. This lighthearted guide to healthful herbal teas includes easy-to-make recipes for the head and throat, digestive system, nervous system, lungs, bones and joints, back, male and female reproductive systems, circulatory system, and skin. Features profiles and favorite recipes from prominent herbalists across North America. Paperback. 160 pages. ISBN 1-58017-099-4.

Henna from Head to Toe! by Norma Pasekoff Weinberg. Body decoration using dyes made from natural henna has never been more popular, and this book offers complete instructions, recipes, and designs for henna skin art. Readers will also find henna recipes for natural hair coloring, nail conditioning, medicinal uses, and more. Hardcover. 80 pages. ISBN 1-58017-097-8.